Let's Talk About Loving

About Love, Sex, Marriage, and Family

Let's Talk About Loving

About Love, Sex, Marriage, and Family

by

Dorothy K. Kripke

and

Myer S. Kripke

Illustrated by
Laszlo Matulay

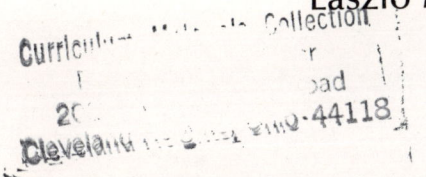

Women's League for Conservative Judaism

KTAV Publishing House, Inc.

Copyright © Dorothy and Myer Kripke 1980

Library of Congress Cataloging in Publication Data

Kripke, Dorothy Karp.
  Let's talk about loving.

  SUMMARY: Discusses, with a Jewish point of view, the different kinds of love—for God, for other people, and, especially and more explicitly, between husbands and wives. Includes chapters on divorce and adoption.
  1. Sex instruction for children. [1. Love.
2. Sex instruction for children. 3. Family life]
I. Kripke, Myer S., joint author. II. Title.
HQ53.K74   306.7   80-22121
ISBN 0-87068-913-4

Manufactured in the United States of America

Contents

To Parents and Teachers 9
Chapter 1—The Many Meanings of Love 13
Chapter 2—How We Recognize Love 17
Chapter 3—Loving God 20
Chapter 4—Loving Yourself 24
Chapter 5—Loving: Parents and Children 28
Chapter 6—Loving: Brothers and Sisters 33
Chapter 7—Loving: The Family 37
Chapter 8—Falling in Love 41
Chapter 9—Male and Female 45
Chapter 10—More About Sex 49
Chapter 11—Loving: Husband and Wife 54
Chapter 12—Not Always—Divorce 60
Chapter 13—Not always—Parents and Children, 64
    Brothers and Sisters
Chapter 14—Not Always—Adoption 69
Chapter 15—The Treasures of Our Hearts 73

Lovingly,
　We dedicate this book to each other
　　and
　　　To Saul and Margaret
　　　To Madeline
　　　To Netta and Yossi

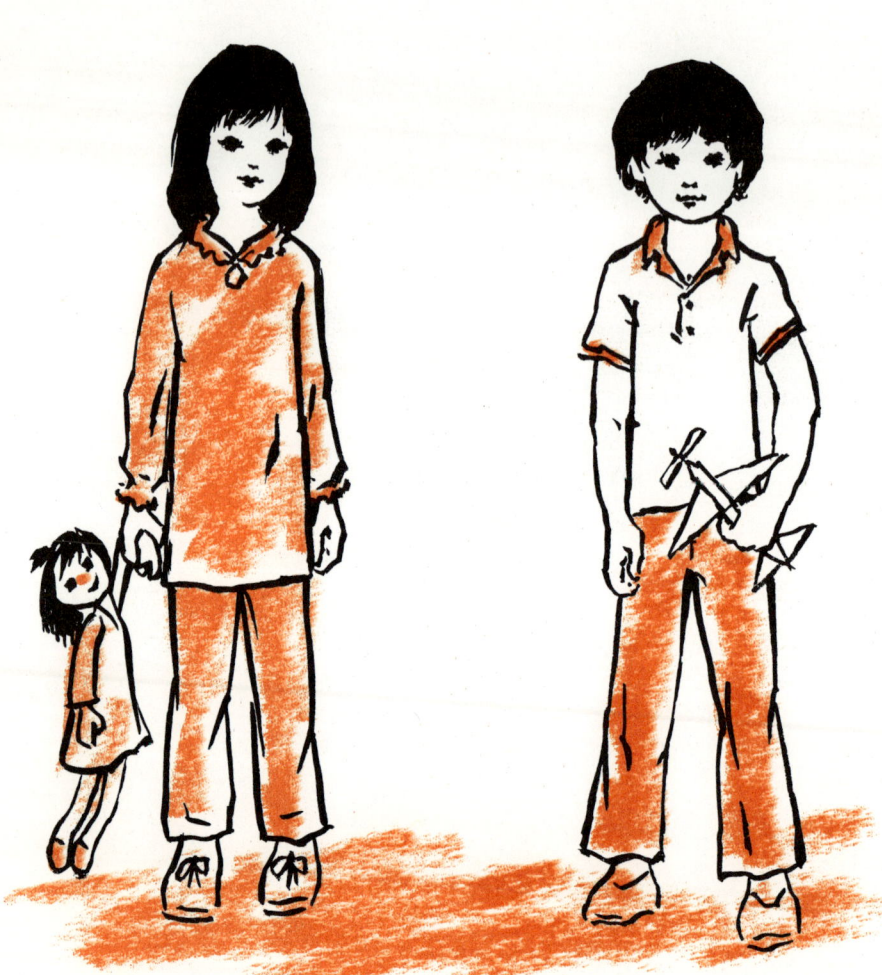

To Parents and Teachers

Early in my work on this book, I felt the need, because of the nature of the subject, for the masculine perspective. Following the example of the masters in the field (on the adult level), who are a husband-and-wife team, I asked my husband to collaborate with me. We hope the result of our collaboration will be of value to both child and parent.

There will be some parents who think we have been too explicit and some who think we have not been explicit enough. Some parents will note that certain subjects are not treated. For various reasons we have omitted them, purposely, relying on the parent to fill in at the proper time.

Basing our judgment on the known natural curiosity of young children, we have tried to tell the child what he/she wants to know and what he/she is capable of comprehending, and to provide a firm and honest foundation for further information. There is an exact spot in the book, moreover, where the alert parent can fill in the simple and obvious answer, implied but not articulated, to the question "How?"—only if it is asked.*

We write from a Jewish religious point of view, which we believe is psychologically sound.

Parents will have to judge the individual child's readiness for this book or any chapter of it. Lest the parent underestimate the young child's interest in the subject and readiness for it, we offer an essay written spontaneously by a bright and well-informed eight-year-old boy, who offered to help his mother with her homework for her college course in Sex Education for Children.

Sex Education for children

God made two sort of human beings ~~on~~ one, Girls and two, boys, now boys and girls both are different boys have penuses and girls have brestes and vagina. And when they Grow up ~~they~~ the boy would be a father and a girl would be a mother. and how to be a mother and a father you have to have a baby and I'll tell you you have a baby it starts out by being sort of a tadpole and there's a millon little tadpoles swimming around her wome and if one gets caut in the wome it will be a baby it takes 9 months for a baby to grow the first two weeks it dosen't look like a baby at all. And all the months of growing he'll start to look like a baby and soon the Mother well get pains and you now what time that is

> time to go to the hospital when you get there, you'll rest for a few days and when comes the nuse will wheel you to the dellevary room and ~~table~~ put, ~~you~~ you on a table the doctor will help broing out. the baby and do all the other things and thats how you get to be a mother and father.

How accurate—and charmingly unselfconscious! Is not this the "consummation devoutly to be wished?"

Dorothy K. Kripke

Omaha, Nebraska

*The "exact spot" is in Chapter 10, "More About Sex," where male and female organs are named and discussed. After you have read " . . . and a boy has a penis through which the sperm is passed to the female," the child may ask "How?" The answer should be delayed, but only slightly, to the point later in the same chapter (next-to-the-last paragraph) where it is said that "husband and wife want to join their lips in kisses and their bodies in an act of love." At this point, in the context of married love, the reading parent, if asked "How?" or "What act of love?" can reply, "During this act of love the male organ enters the female organ and releases the sperm." Now the reading parent can continue with the text itself, "And it is then, some of the time, that the male sperm finds the female ovum, so that a new life begins."

The parent, of course, may want to express it differently. But since many parents find this question difficult to handle, we offer the above as a simple, direct, and honest answer.

D.K.K   M.S.K.

Chapter 1

The Many Meanings of Love

Do you remember an amusing conversation about words in *Through the Looking-Glass,* that Alice has with Humpty Dumpty? "That's a great deal to make one word mean," Alice said.

"When I make a word do a lot of work like that," said Humpty Dumpty, "I always pay it extra."

In this conversation (and throughout that delightful book), the author is playing with words. He is having fun; and the reader has fun along with him. But he is making a point: that some words have many meanings.

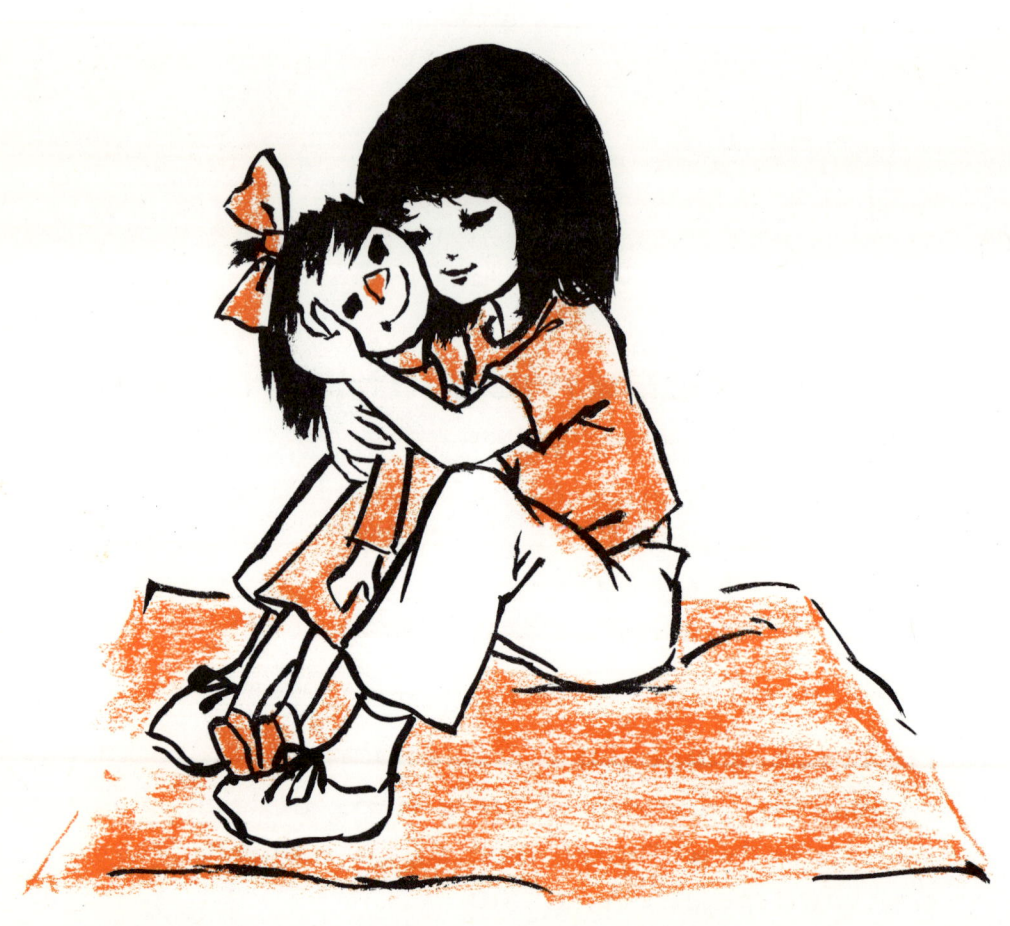

If we think about the word "playing," we see how many jobs it does, how many meanings it has. People play games, like hide-and-seek and checkers and cards. In sports, we say we are playing baseball or football or tennis. On the stage or screen, an actor is playing a role. Both the actor and the audience know that the actor is only pretending. We know he is not really Abraham Lincoln or the Wizard of Oz. But the actor tries to play his part so that this "make-believe" seems real. The magician "plays tricks" on his audience. He pulls a rabbit out of his hat, or a string of scarfs, red and yellow and blue and green, and tries to fool us into thinking it is really magic. People play the piano, the violin, the flute—or even records.

Humpty Dumpty will certainly have to pay a lot extra, won't he?

In the same way, the word "loving" has many meanings. Loving God means recognizing His work in the world, appreciating it—and more. Loving ourselves means self-respect—and more. Loving our neighbors means fairness to all people, whether we know them or not. Love of parents for children means sharing and responsibility and guidance and protection—and respect. Love of children for parents means respect—and much more. Loving one's brothers and sisters means sharing and helping. Loving one's country and one's people means loyalty and protection and obeying the laws. Love of a man and a woman, a husband and wife, for each other means all of these and even more, much more. When a husband and a wife truly love each other, their love is special and full of joy.

In all of these cases, loving means "caring." When we care for someone we mean, "You are very dear to me. You are a very important part of my life. What happens to you is important to me."

Now let's look at the different kinds of loving and try to understand the many meanings of love.

Chapter 2

How We Recognize Love

We cannot see love. And yet we recognize it by what it does to us, by the way it makes us feel. It makes us feel warm and safe and comfortable. Deep inside ourselves, without words and without melody, our whole being sings a song of joy. Love makes us happy.

When we love we want to please, to help, to protect, to share with those we love. We want to share not only things, but our work, our time, our feelings, our thoughts, ourselves. We want to be fair and honest. We care for those we love and as far as possible want to take care of them.

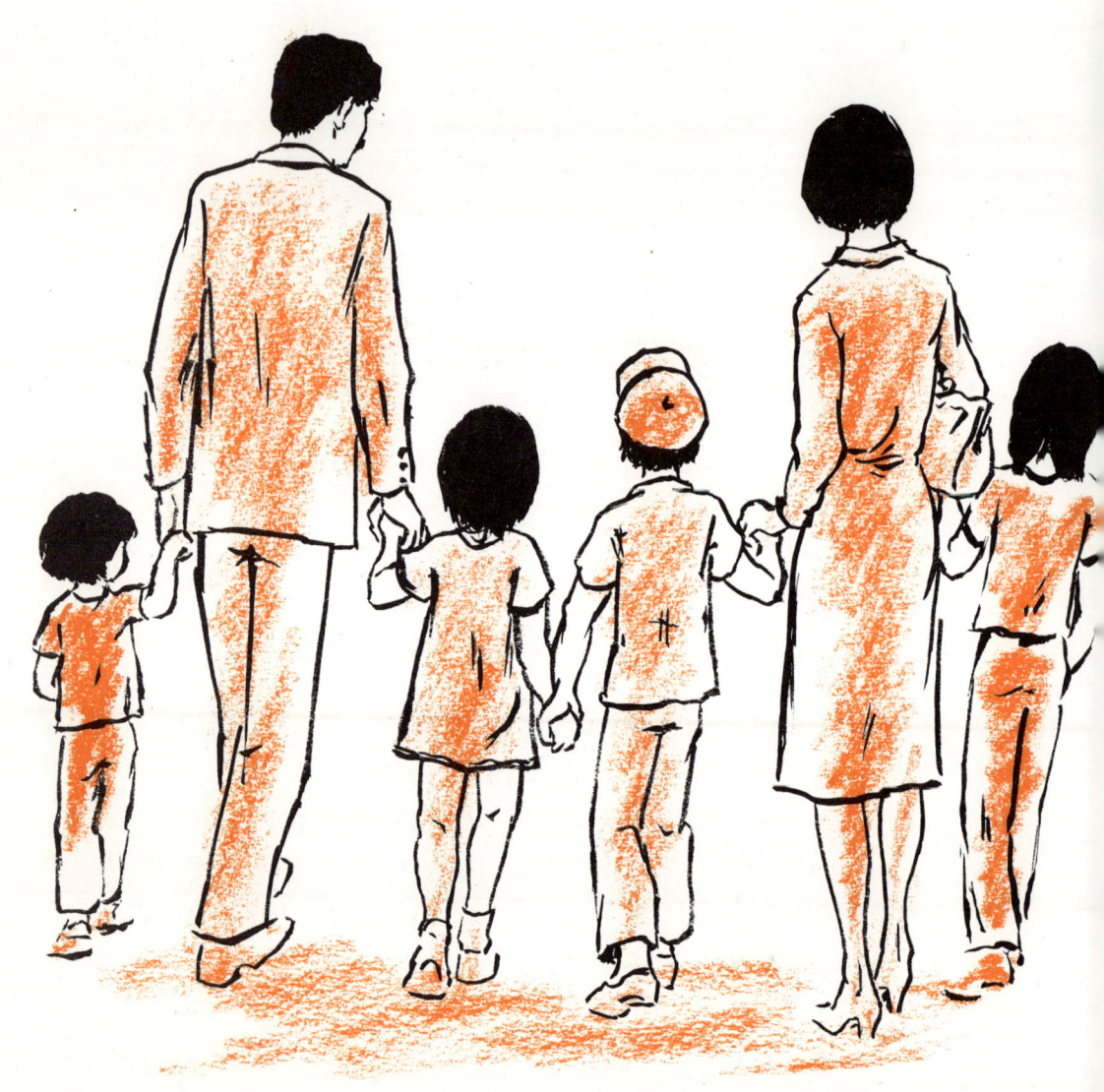

When we are loved, we feel safe and protected. We feel comfortable with those who love us. We can be ourselves, with no pretending. We feel love in a hug, a kiss, an arm about our shoulders. We know it in a squeeze, a touch, a loving look—even in a wink. Being loved makes us feel happy with ourselves, and glad to be alive. It makes us want to share our joys and pleasures. It makes us able to share our disappointments and sorrows. Then, in sad times we feel a little comforted. In happy times our joy seems to sparkle all the more.

We all need to love. And we all need to be loved. Love makes us appreciate life more, enjoy it more, value it more. We are not alone; love makes us feel we belong to each other.

Chapter 3

Loving God

Later on in this book, we shall talk about the love of a boy and a girl (or a man and a woman) for each other. This is a special kind of loving. To understand how this kind of love fits into the pattern of our lives, we need to talk about other kinds of loving first.

The Bible tells us to love God. What does it mean to love God? How do we do it? First of all, we must understand that there is one God in all the

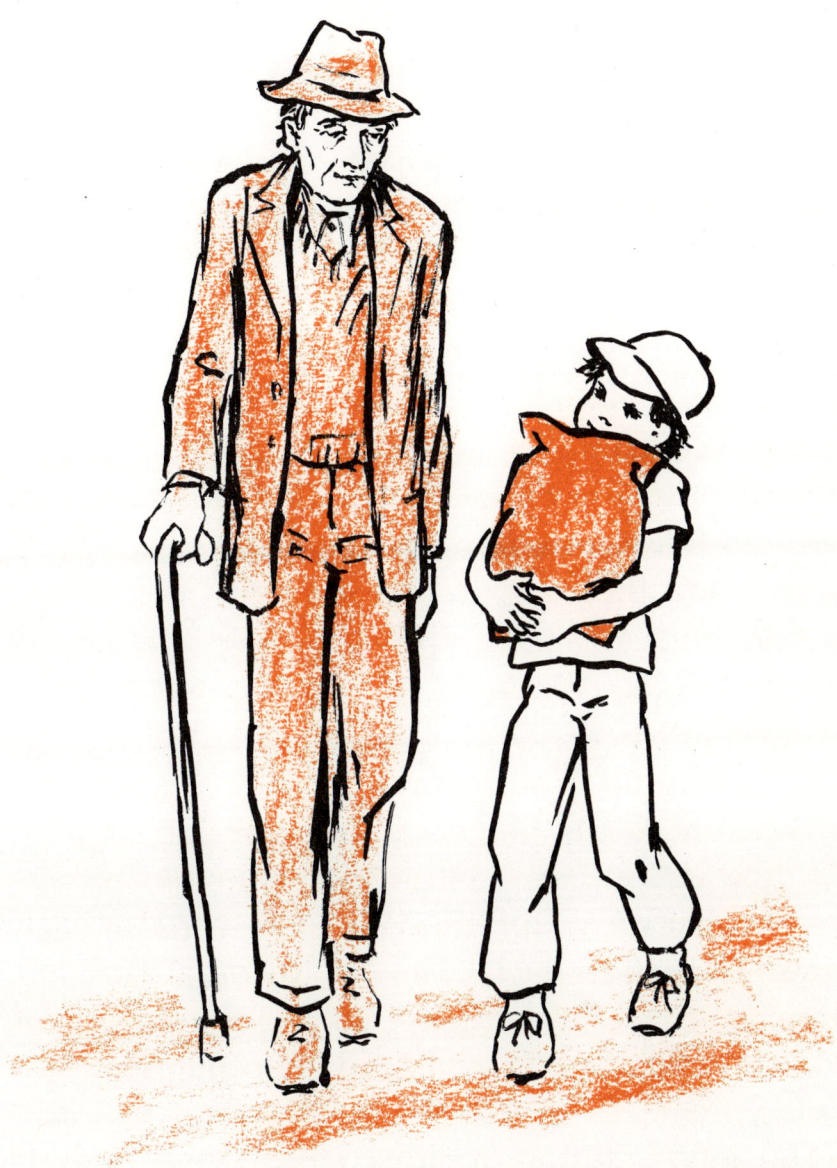

world. He may be called by different names, but there is only one God. The whole world is His, the earth on which we live and all that it contains. The planets, the stars in their courses, the whirling galaxies, all, all these too are His, and the vastness of outer space in which they move.

We show our love for God by appreciating His world, by caring for it, by using it well, by being careful not to spoil or hurt or damage or pollute it. You may have heard or read about conservation or ecology. We use these words to remind us that air and water and other treasures of the earth must be used carefully, and not destroyed. We, or our children and their children, will need them later on. And from a religious point of view it is even more than that: We must not destroy what God has made for us.

All the people in the world are His. We are all His children. All people, no matter who they are or how they look or where they live, are children of God. We can show our love of God by the way we treat all His children.

How should we treat them? The Bible gives us an important clue. It tells us, "Love your neighbor as yourself." This idea, translated from three simple Hebrew words, is one of the most important ideas in the world. Two thousand years ago it became the basis for Hillel's Golden Rule. Rabbi Akiba called it "The Great Rule of the Torah." Let's think about the three parts of this Great Rule to see exactly what it means.

What does "your neighbor" mean? It means any other (and every other) person in the world. "But," you will argue, "I don't even know every person in the world!" That is exactly the point. The Bible tells us to love even the people we don't know, the anonymous people.

But, you may be thinking, there are some people you don't even like. How can you love them? Or the anonymous people, the ones you don't even know? Now we come to a new meaning of love, a new understanding of loving. Loving here means *being fair*. And we can be fair to people whom we don't know. And we can be fair even to people we don't like. "Love your neighbor as yourself" really means, "Be as fair to all people everywhere as to yourself." When we treat all people fairly, we are showing God that we love Him. Fairness, justice, is a way of loving God.

We have said that "Love" in the Great Rule means "Be fair." And "your neighbor" means "all people." We have not yet talked about the third part, "as yourself." Let's do that in the next chapter.

Chapter 4

Loving Yourself

Sometimes the earth's treasures are on the surface, right on top where we can see them, like fields of wheat and grain, or orchards of fruit trees. Sometimes the treasure is hidden deep in the earth, like diamonds and gold and coal and oil. We must dig deep to find them. Ideas are like that too. Sometimes they are clear on the surface; and sometimes we must dig deep for the treasure of hidden meanings.

The meaning of "Love your neighbor as yourself" is like that. Part of it is very clear. It means

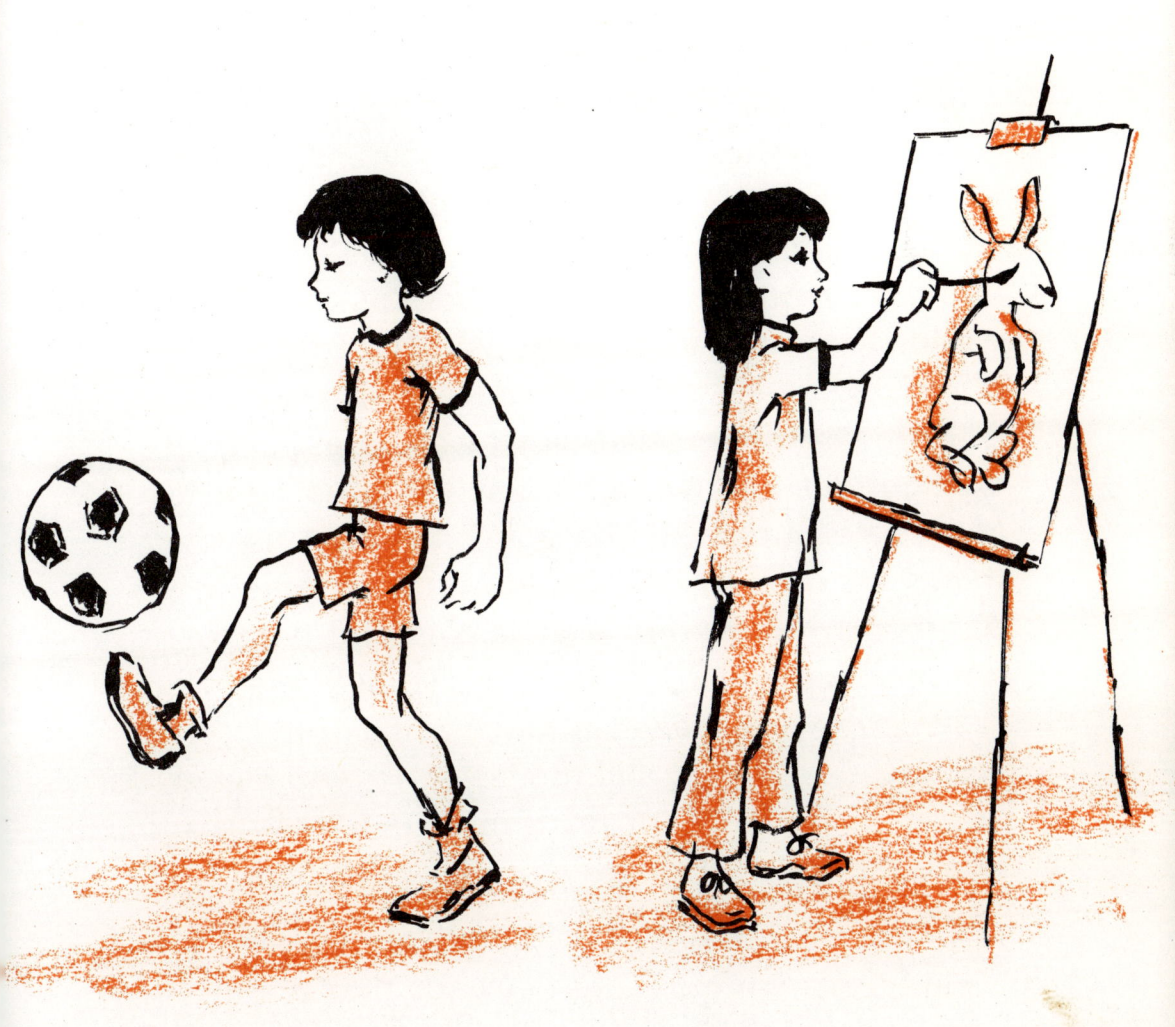

"Be as fair to all people as you are to yourself."

There is also a hidden meaning. "As yourself" means "as you love yourself." This tells us, "Love yourself. Be fair to yourself."

Taken together, the clear meaning and the hidden meaning tell us: Every other person in the world is important—and so are you. You are important—but so is every other person in the world. We must love them. And we must love ourselves.

In the case of ourselves, loving includes liking. It is important that we like ourselves. It is right to appreciate ourselves, the good that is in us, the things we do well. We try to improve ourselves, our minds, our bodies, our talents. But we must not be disappointed if there are some things we can't improve or change as much as we would like.

Someone else may still run faster or jump higher or play piano better or learn math more easily or sing better or be stronger or prettier than you.

Still, there is one thing *you* do best. No one can be better at it than you. And that is being yourself and being the best "you" you can! No one else in the whole world is you. And it is right that you accept yourself. You try hard to be as special a "you" as possible, as bright or as strong or as pretty as possible. Then be content to be as you are. God's world is full of variety, and you—and every other person—are part of that variety.

The wonderful thing about that variety is that although we are all different from each other, in one way we are all alike. We are all different because some of us are one color, some another; some of us are male, some female; we live in different places of the world and speak different languages. Even so, we are all alike because there is a little bit of God in every human being. This is what the Bible means when it tells us that we are made "in the image of God." That is why each of us is important, each of us special, you and I and everyone else. And that is why we owe ourselves self-respect. And that is why we must respect every other person.

> Loving ourselves means being fair to ourselves and liking ourselves, at the same time remembering that we are to love other people and be fair to them too.

Chapter 5

Loving: Parents and Children

At the beginning of this book we said that love has many meanings. And we said that one of these meanings is the respect between children and parents.

But love for our parents is much, much more than that, so much more that it can hardly be explained. Later in this book we will learn that our parents have given us our lives and even our bodies. They loved us and cared for us and watched over us even before we were born. Before we were born—and after.

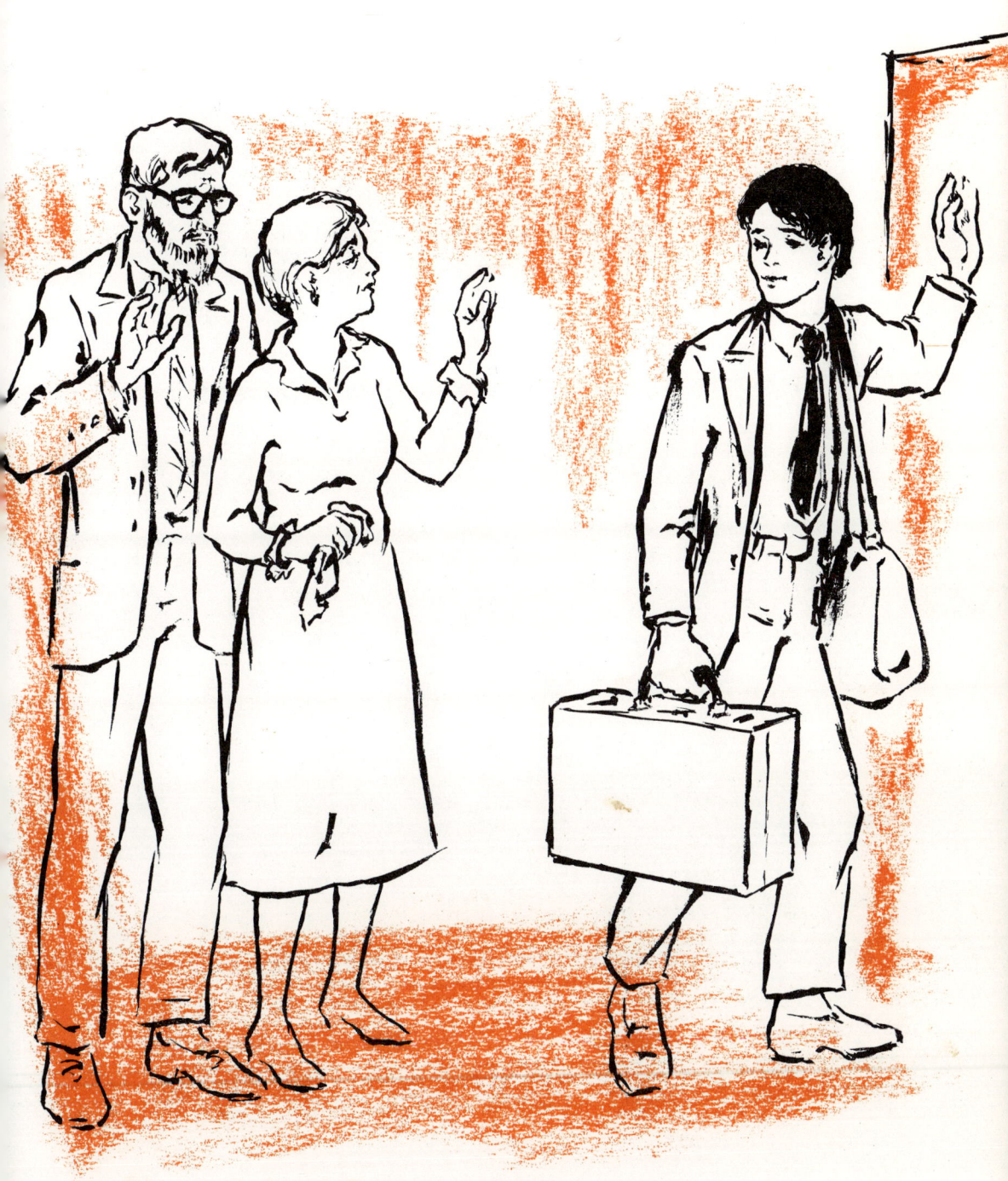

Have you ever seen a tiny newborn baby sleeping, so peaceful, so beautiful, so trusting—and so helpless? We were all that way once. Our parents gave us food even before we knew how to ask for it. Before we knew how to do anything for ourselves, they kept us warm and clean. They tried to guard us against illness and accident. They helped us learn to hold a spoon, to walk, to ride a bike, to grow up. All this is part of love.

There is a kind of chain of love. Your parents got love from their parents and gave it to you. And you will one day pass it on to your children, and in time they will pass it on to theirs.

And the chain is not all one way, from parents to children. It goes in the other direction too, from children to parents. There is a magic to love that is hard to explain. It can only be felt. The magic is that just as our fathers and mothers give us their love, we feel love for them. It fills our hearts and minds. Our whole spirit, our whole self loves them.

We can do many things for our parents. We love them in as many ways as we can, and try to please them in any way we can. In some families, a time comes when parents need their children's help. Then loving children help as much as they can. There is a magic in the love between parents and children, a love that we share in the most natural way possible, as naturally as we breathe, without thinking about it, as naturally as we think and see and hear.

How do we show love for our parents? Not only by wanting to be with them and by hugs and kisses. We show it by respecting them and their opinions and their teaching. We may not always agree with them. But we know that they love us and that nothing makes them happier than when good things happen to us. So we listen to their ideas with respect and think of their advice carefully. While we are young we try to do what they ask us to do. We try to be loving and obedient sons and daughters. We listen to our parents and respect them.

One day, when we are old enough, we will have to make decisions for ourselves. Our fathers and mothers understand this. This, indeed, is what our parents have been trying to do all along: to help us do things for ourselves, to think for ourselves, to become independent! This is what growing up means. We will be responsible for ourselves.

Sometimes this gets pretty complicated, all mixed up. Our parents want us to learn to make our own decisions; and yet they can't keep from making suggestions that sound as though they are telling us what to do! They are trying to help us. And at the same time they are trying to help us grow up. That's why it seems so mixed up.

But we will still listen to our parents and honor and respect them. Even when we make our own decisions, we will still consider their advice very carefully, whether we follow it or not. Our love for them is forever.

Loving parents respect their children too. They listen to their children and try to understand what they *really* mean in what they say and what they do. Since no one is perfect, there are times when parents do not understand. And there are times when children make mistakes. In spite of this, the magic of their love remains. The love of parents and children for each other is forever.

Another way of saying all this is that children are people and parents are people. People with needs of their own, rights of their own, problems of their own, mistakes of their own—lives of their own. Understanding this (and remembering it!) is an important part of the love of parents and children for each other.

Chapter 6

Loving: Brothers and Sisters

The love within a family—parents and children, brothers and sisters—is very special. What, you may be asking, is so special about brothers and sisters? Think of this:

No one in the whole world—except your brothers and sisters—has the same parents, the same grandparents, and the same home, as you. They are the only ones who grow up with you, eat the same food at the same table, and share the love of the same parents. They are more like you than any other person in the whole world. You

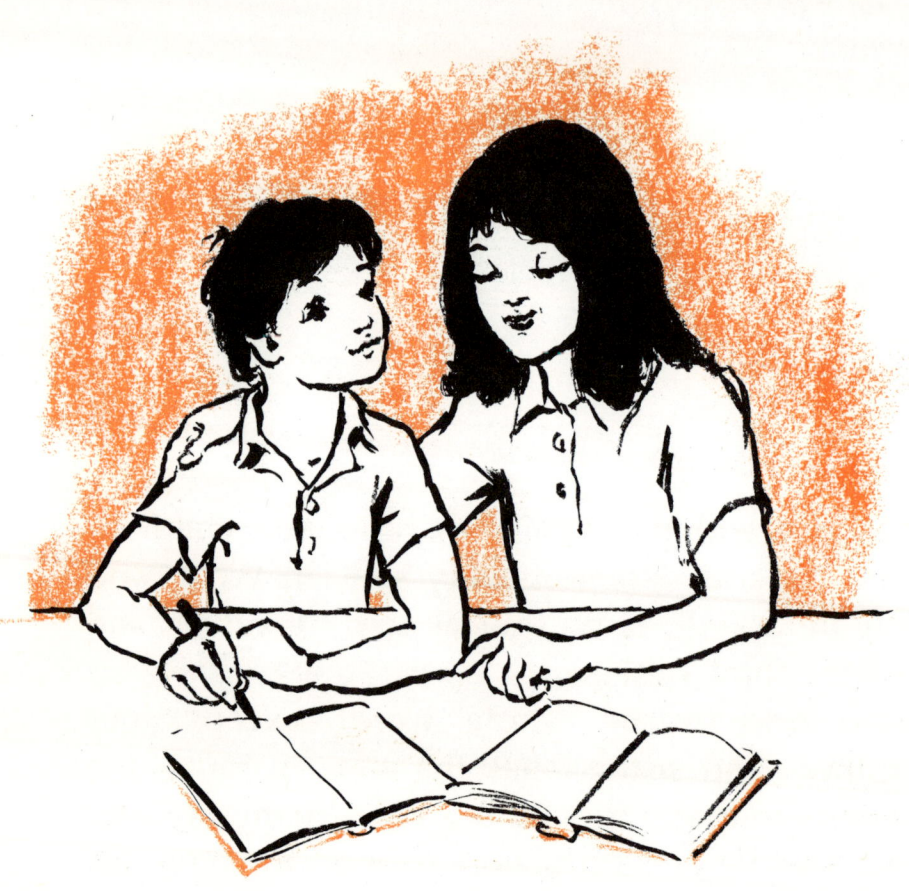

may even look alike. Or sound alike. Later, when you study science, you will learn why you look alike, and why your bodies and your minds are alike in many important ways. Together you are brothers and sisters, children of the same parents.

As we grow older, we make friends with other people. We meet other children at school. Or there are other children who are neighbors. And they become our friends. Some of these friendships last our whole life through, and they are very precious. Friends who are real friends will do wonderful things for each other. They are very close to each other, sometimes as close as brothers and sisters. They love each other.

But usually brothers and sisters care for each other even more than friends. They have lived together in one home. They have shared the experiences of growing up together; they have shared in the love of the same parents; they have had good times together. As they grow older they have memories of things they did together as a family. There were picnics, perhaps, and family celebrations and holidays, and summer vacations and trips. They shared many things. And the more we share, the more we feel we belong to each other.

Even though they may quarrel (as they often do!), sisters and brothers belong to each other and love one another.

When you are older and have a home of your own, just like your brothers and sisters, you will realize how good it is to know that they are there and that you can always count on them. And they can count on you. They love you, just as you love them.

Chapter 7

Loving: The Family

The people we have just been talking about—parents and children, brothers and sisters—are a *family*.

You knew that, of course. But you probably never thought about it before.

Your best friend may eat with your family now and then and perhaps stay overnight with you. In return, you may visit your friend's family and stay overnight, or even for a few days. What fun this is! But that's only now and then. Your friend goes home. You come back to your family. Usually, you and your family are together.

You are with them so much, your parents and brothers and sisters, that your family is your first teacher! Did you ever think about that? Your family is a teacher that never has to tell you, "Now we are going to have a lesson." The lessons in the family are learned without ever having to say, "Now here is something for us to learn." The learning in the family is simply from living together.

The most important thing you learn in your family is what love is. Members of a family love each other, give themselves to each other, do things for each other, are fair with each other, without ever having to think about it.

And, in your family, you learn how to get along with other people. Without thinking about it! Members of your family are people too—and just as you expect them to be responsible and reliable, they expect you to be responsible and reliable. And honest and fair. And helpful. And loving. You belong to the people in your family in a special way; and in the same way they belong to you.

If you are lucky enough to have grandparents and cousins and aunts and uncles, you know that they are part of your family too. This is because

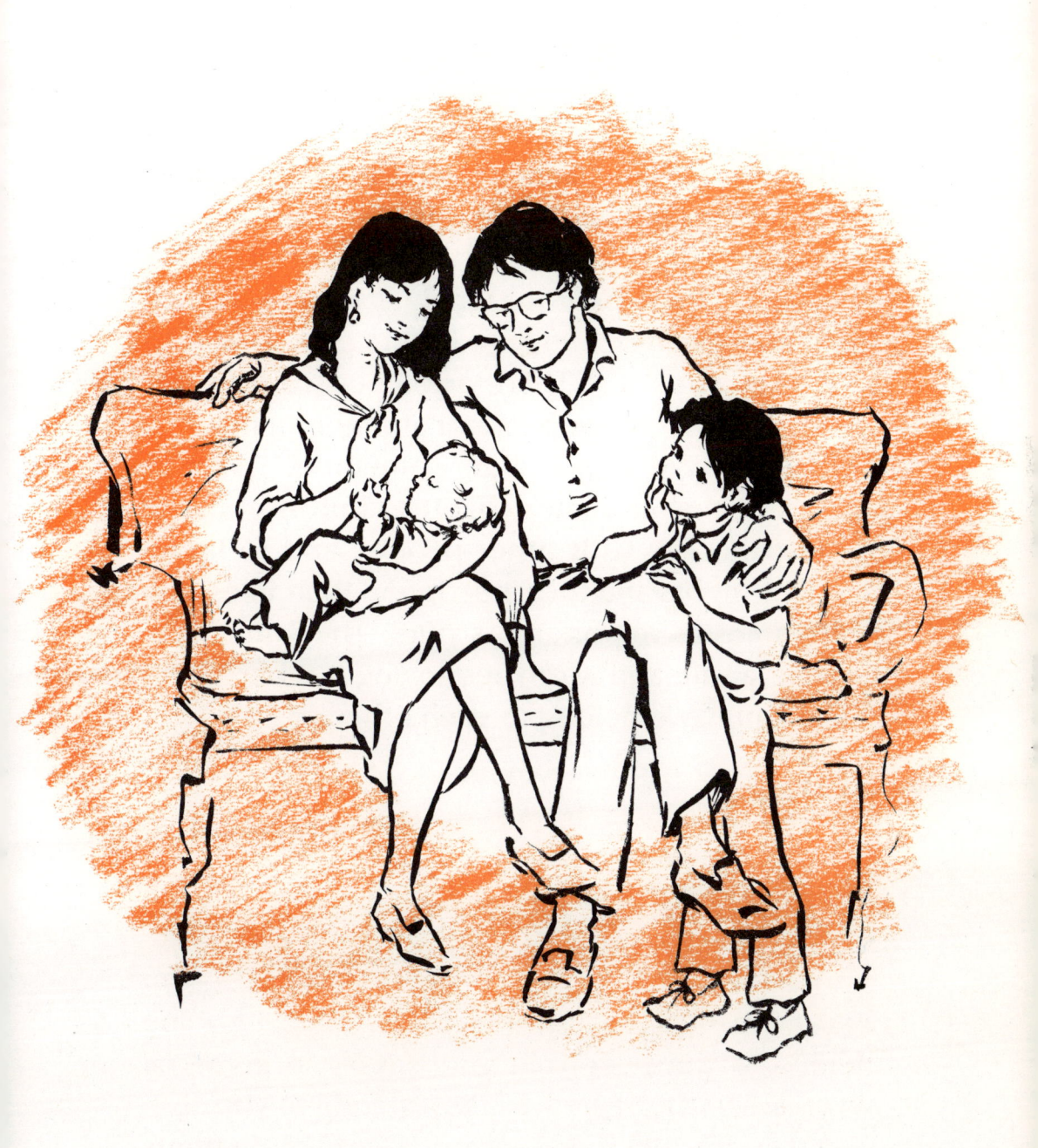

your father, when he was a boy, had a family—and all the people in his family are part of your family. And your mother, when she was a girl, had a family too—and they are all part of your family too.

It is good to be part of a family. It is here that we learn how to enjoy the love others give us and to give love ourselves. There are times, to be sure, when we are angry with one or another member of our family. (We all get angry sometimes! We will talk about this in a later chapter.) But this is how we learn to live with other people, and to know that their rights and their needs and their likes and dislikes are as important as ours. The family is a teacher, a safe and warm and loving teacher.

In a family we belong to each other.

Chapter 8

Falling in Love

Why is it that a home usually has a father and mother? Why did they make a home together? Each of them once had a home in which he was the child, in which she was the child. Why is it that when they grew up, he and she wanted to be husband and wife, wanted to have children, wanted to be father and mother?

You can be told the answer to these questions even when you are young. But you will not really understand the answer until you are older, and can *feel* the answer yourself.

The answer tells us about one of the most wonderful things in life. While we are young, boys usually like to play with boys, and girls with girls. At the same time, boys want to know about girls, and girls want to know about boys. Then, when we grow older, there is something we can't explain, something within us, something we feel, that makes a boy like to be with a girl, and makes a girl like to be with a boy. It is as though a powerful magnet draws them together, a magnet you cannot see. It is the magnet of sex.

And each of them feels good. A girl feels good to be with a boy. And a boy feels good to be with a girl.

This is the beginning of a new kind, a different kind, of love. While he grows through the years till he is a man, a boy may have several friends who are girls; and a girl may have several friends who are boys during her growing years. But one day the girl will find one boy, and the boy will find one girl, who seems to be the best person in all the world. A boy and a girl who have found each other and feel that way about each other, who think that the other is the best person in the world, want to be with each other always. They want to spend their whole life together. They want to be husband and wife to each other. They are in love.

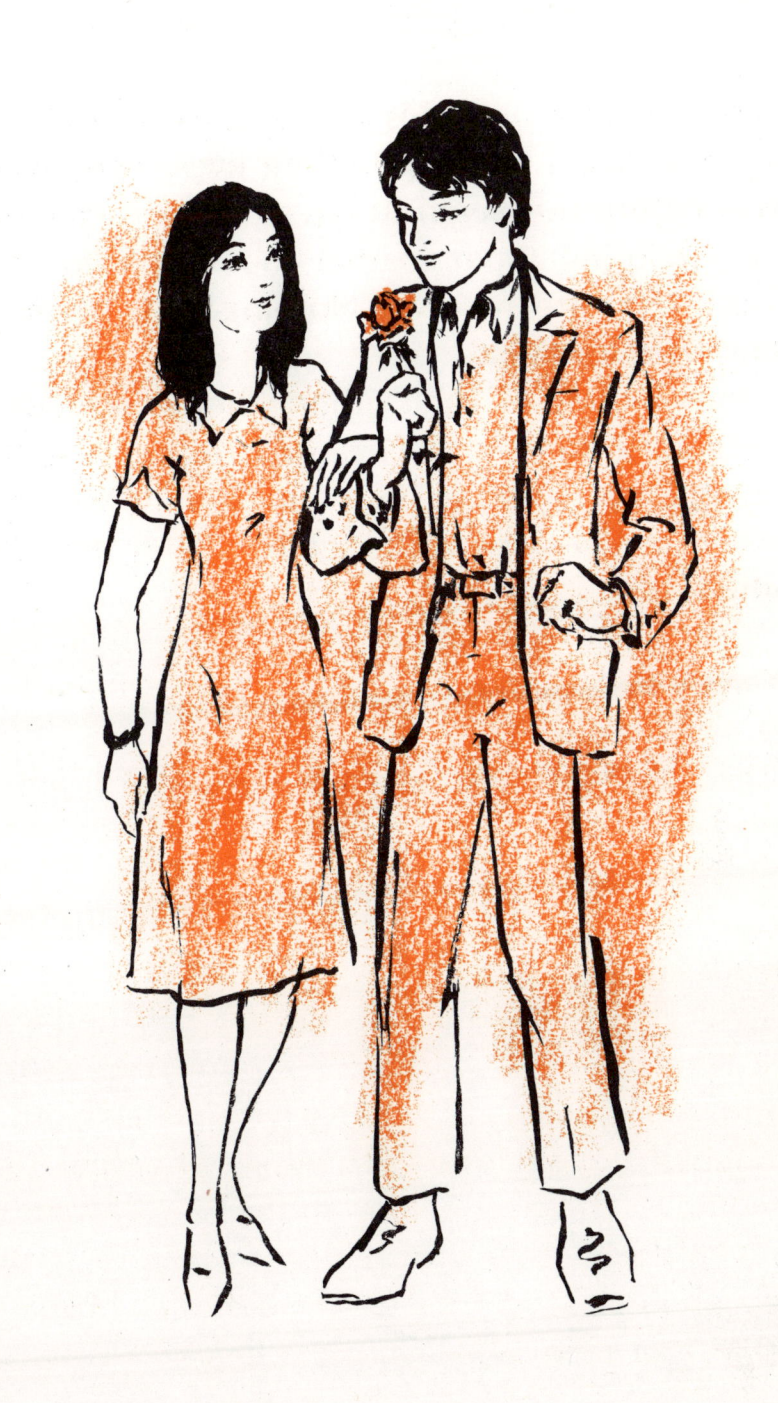

When they realize this and say it to each other, it is the happiest moment in their lives. Their whole lives before this seem to have had one main reason, to bring them to that moment when they know they are in love. Nothing else seems so important to them.

They belong to each other. They will enjoy all the good things of life even more, because they are together. And the hard things of life will seem easier, because they are together. They love each other.

Chapter 9

Male and Female

We have already talked about a boy and a girl who want to be together forever because they are in love with each other.

But this is so strange! Here we have two people who probably did not even know each other during their childhood years! And yet, when they meet and spend some time together as a grown boy and a grown girl (or man and woman), they decide that they want to be together always!

What pulls them together? What is this magnet between the sexes?

You have surely noticed that boys and girls look different. When they are grown up, boys usually, but not always, are taller than girls, and heavier. Their muscles are heavier too. So they are stronger. And most girls are shorter and lighter than most boys, and usually they are not so strong. Their bodies have more curves than boys', gentle curves.

But these differences are not the main ones that make boys and men males, and girls and women females. Both males and females have wonderful parts to their bodies, but the male parts and the female parts are different from each other.

The female body is so wonderful that a tiny baby can grow inside it until the baby is ready to be born. Before its birth the baby gets all it needs from its mother, food and shelter and everything else, until its own parts—heart and lungs and all—can work all by themselves, outside the mother's body. Then it is born.

A male cannot carry a baby inside his body. Only the female can carry the baby. But the baby's life cannot begin without the male. There is a female life-part and a male life-part which join together. That is why a baby has a father and a mother. Both male and female are necessary. The father is the

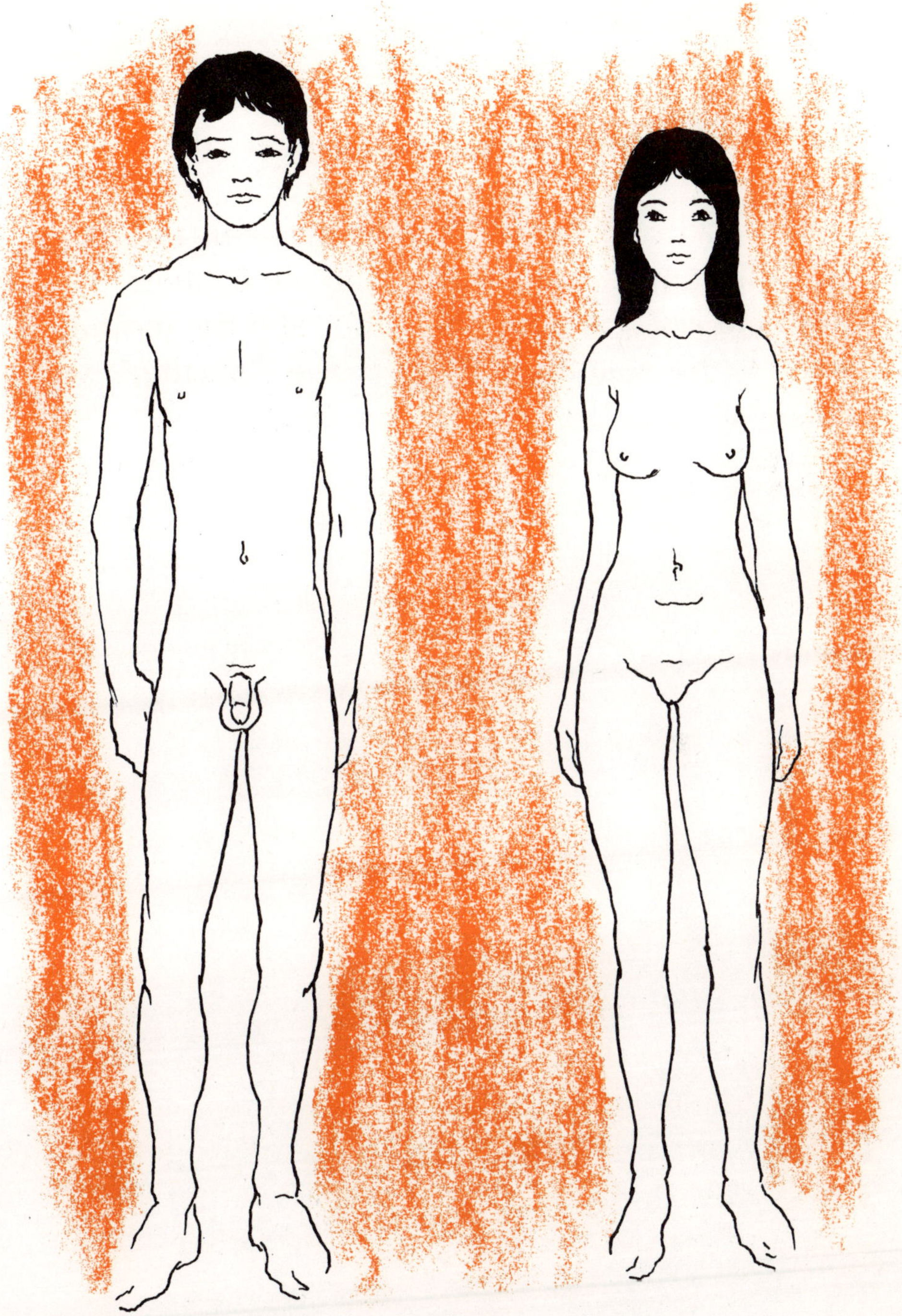

male. The mother is the female. Men and boys are the male sex; and women and girls are the female sex.

We shall never really know why—but the male and the female want to be with each other. The husband and the wife, the father and the mother, want to be together. (That is the "magnet" we talked about!) They love each other.

Chapter 10

More About Sex

We have learned some of the differences between boys and girls, and the differences between the male sex and the female sex.

Male and female together start the nine-month process of a new life, when the male and the female life-parts join together. Then, for nine months, the female nourishes a baby inside her own body. We say that the woman is *pregnant*. She is going to have a baby.

What are the life-parts which join together to start a baby growing inside the mother?

The male life-part is the *sperm,* and the female life-part is the *ovum.* When the two meet, the sperm and the ovum, the miracle of a new life begins. Both the sperm and the ovum are very tiny. They are so tiny that they cannot be seen without a microscope.

When we are old enough, usually around ten or twelve or fourteen, our bodies begin to produce the male and female life-parts. This happens because we have *sex organs.* "Organs" are parts of the body, like eyes and ears, like the heart and the lungs. The organs that make us male or female are called sex organs.

The lower part of the body, which rests on the legs, is called the pelvis. Most of the sex organs, together with other organs, are in the pelvis or near it. A boy's sex organs are mostly on the outside of the body, and a girl's mostly inside.

A boy has testicles, which produce the male life-part, the sperm; and a boy has a penis, through which the sperm is passed to the female.

A girl has a hollow organ, called a vagina. It starts from an opening into the body. At the other end, inside the body, are other sex organs. One of these produces the ovum. Another is the uterus, or womb. The womb is marvelously made for a baby to grow in, from its tiniest beginning until it is ready to be born.

FEMALE SEX ORGAN

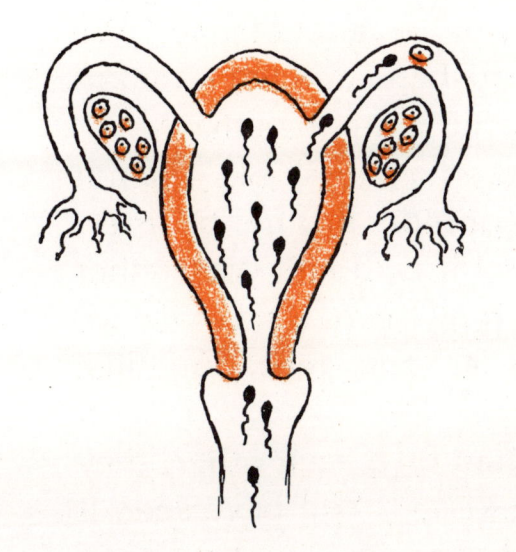

MALE SEX ORGAN

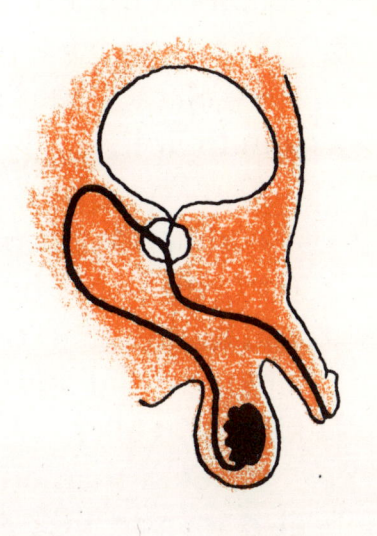

A girl also has breasts. When she is old enough, her breasts begin to grow and give her chest a beautiful shape, soft and rounded. Nature, in its marvelous way, is preparing the girl for the time, much later, when she will be a mother. For nine months, while a baby is growing in the womb, it gets its food from inside the mother's body. Then, when the baby is born, the miracle of life fills the mother's breasts with sweet warm milk, the perfect food for a newborn baby.

Let us go back now to our "magnet of love." We have already said that a husband and wife want to join their lives. But it is even more than that.

You know how contented a baby looks when it is cuddled by its parents or older brother or sister. And you know how sweet it is to kiss your father and mother and be kissed by them. (Of course we all know that some boys, at some ages, don't like kissing at all!)

When a man and woman love each other, they also love to kiss and be kissed. You have seen it many times on TV or in the movies. You have seen your mother and father kissing. But a husband and wife have other caresses, and other acts of love, so tender that they are very private. A husband and wife want to join their lips in kisses and their bodies in an act of love. And it is then, some of the time, that the male sperm finds the female ovum, so that a new life begins. This is the way that the life of each of us began. Even the lives of our parents! Even our grandparents!

It is here that we reach into the holiest powers that God has given us. We have already said that He gave us male and female bodies. And now we add that our sex powers make it possible for us to share in the miracle of starting a new life.

Chapter 11

Loving: Husband and Wife

In an earlier chapter, we tried to understand why a boy and a girl, or a man and a woman, fall in love. We tried to understand. But we never really could!

We didn't understand because we can't really tell why this man and that woman fall in love with each other—only with each other and not with someone else!

This is the "magic of love." It is "magic" because the strong attraction between a man and a woman *is* there—and yet it is something we can't really explain.

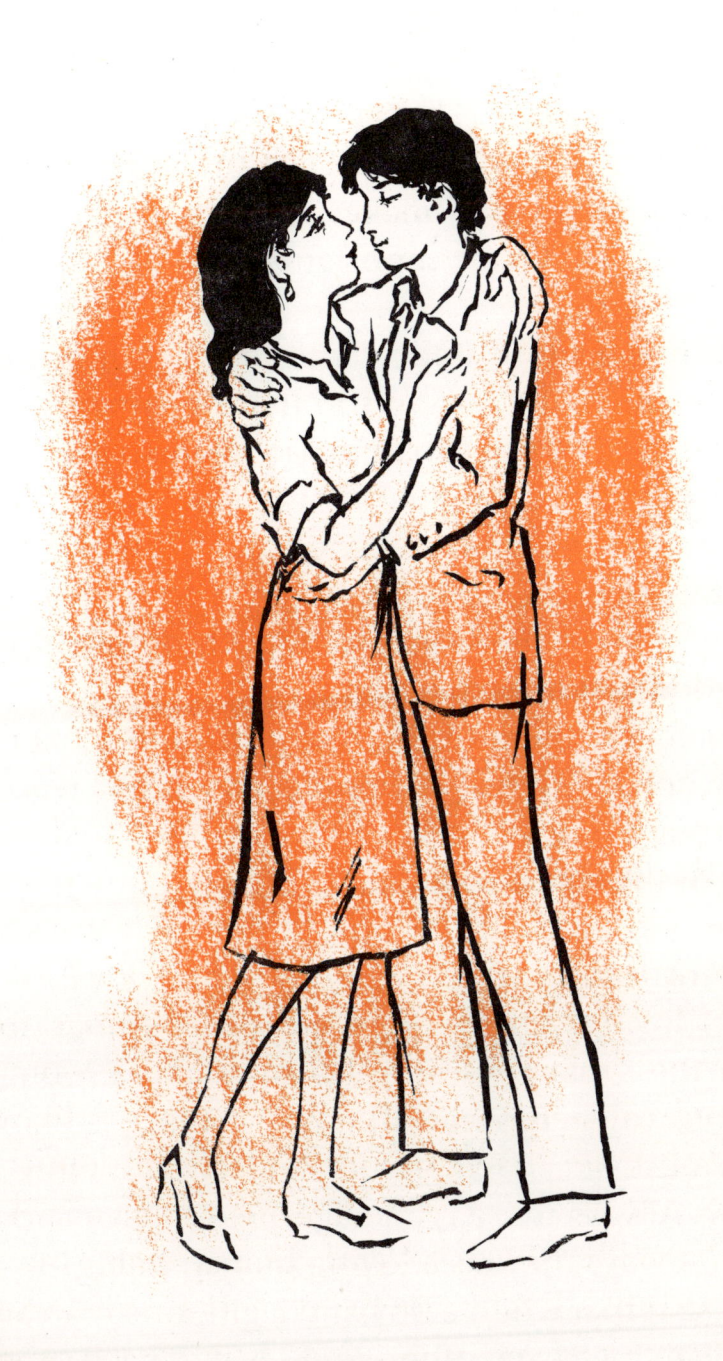

You might think, because we have talked so much about sex and sex organs that it is only the attraction of sex that makes a woman and a man fall in love. That is an important part of it. But there is much more.

There is a more important part. The more important part is the *real person* that a woman is, and the *real person* that a man is. The woman seems to the man to be just the kind of person he wants to be with. It makes him feel good just to be near her. And the man seems to the woman to be just the kind of person she wants to be with. It makes her feel good just to be near him.

Usually we think of the real person in a man as one who is strong, yet gentle and kind, who is generous and loyal, and always loving. Usually we think of the real person in a woman as one who is gentle and kind, but strong in her own ways, in different ways, who is generous and loyal, and always loving. Often there are other things that make the "real person" of a man and a woman precious to each other. But always there is liking. They must *like* each other. And always there is loyalty. Always there is an eagerness to give and to share. Always there is a loving human being.

We said that when a boy and a girl, or a man and a woman, love each other, and say it to each other, their happiness is so great that it seems that all their lives have been leading to that moment. Yet there is another moment more important even than that. It is the time of the wedding.

Loving each other, they have said that they would marry, that they would be husband and wife to each other. Then there is a wedding. Sometimes the wedding is small, with only a few people. Sometimes it is large, with many relatives and friends who share in the happiness of bride and bridegroom, of wife and husband. A marriage is so important that people in every part of the world and in all times have considered it important not only to bride and groom, but also to everyone around them, to society. A rabbi joins the bride and bridegroom in marriage. Always it is reported to the government, so that all may know that this man and woman are married. They are husband and wife.

A man and a woman think of their marriage, when they became husband and wife, as the most important and the happiest thing that has ever happened to them. Because they love each other, they now share their lives. They live in one home, together. The money they earn usually belongs to both of them, together. They spend their time together. Of course each may like to have some time alone or to spend with friends; but most of the time, when they are not at work, they like to be together. Everything, everything is together.

They are two separate people, of course. He is himself, with his own likes and dislikes. She is herself, with her own special likes and dislikes. But they understand each other and are willing for their differences to be. Even with the differences, they love each other.

We know that husbands and wives love to kiss each other and embrace each other, to hold each other close in a loving hug. Sometimes they join their bodies as well as their lips. It is one of the sweetest things in life to be husband and wife in this way. It is the special loving of husband and wife. It is good and full of joy.

And sometimes this married love, as we have said in an earlier chapter, leads to forming another life, a tiny baby.

Husband and wife are very special to each other. Their love is one of the most precious things in their life together, and it makes everything in life more important and more meaningful. If they have troubles, they know that carrying them together makes the hurt a little easier to bear. And when they have special joys, like a new baby, their joy is deeper and stronger because of their love for each other.

Husband and wife expect to be special to each other all through their lives. Each of them, the husband and the wife, may certainly have friends of the other sex. But not in the way that married people are special friends and lovers, husband and wife, to each other. Husband and wife belong to each other, and only to each other. They trust each other. The husband knows that his wife gives herself only to him. And the wife knows that her husband gives himself only to her.

They are faithful to each other. Their love is for each other—and they want it to be so forever.

Chapter 12

Not Always—Divorce

Most of us know the story of the princess and the frog. Her kiss breaks the wicked spell and turns the frog back into a prince. There are stories, too, of the prince whose kiss wakes the girl from sleep or turns her into a princess. In these stories, there may be hidden meanings. (Do you remember that we talked about hidden meanings in an earlier chapter?) These hidden meanings may be telling us something about real life. To the boy in love, one particular girl seems like a princess. To the girl in love, one special boy seems like her prince. The

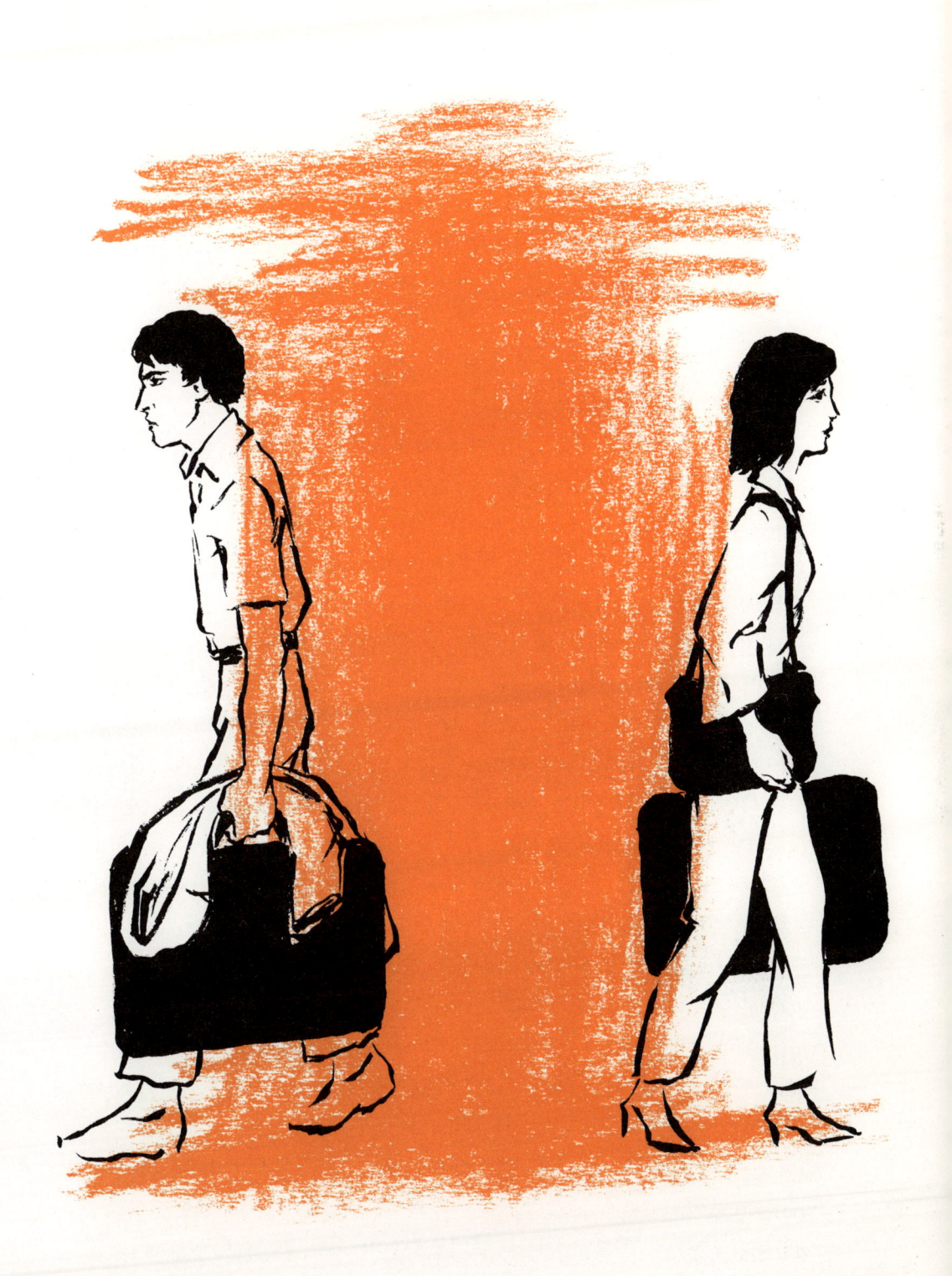

boy who is loved feels like a prince; and the girl who is loved feels like a princess. In these stories the prince and princess get married. The stories end by telling us "and they lived happily ever after."

But in real life, the living-happily-ever-after is not always so.

A man and a woman are ready for marriage only when they are quite grown up. Not only in their bodies, but also in their thinking and their understanding of real life. If they expect marriage to take them into fairyland or an enchanted castle, where everything will be perfect, they are expecting the impossible. They are not ready for marriage. Real life has illnesses and accidents, as well as pleasures and happiness and joy. People who are really grown-up understand that they must expect at least some of the bad things as well as the good. If they expect marriage to be one long birthday party, with cake and ice cream and presents wrapped in pretty paper and tied with a ribbon, they will be disappointed.

Sometimes a husband and wife are disappointed in each other. This can happen even to two good people. Perhaps they are just not a good combination—like pickles and ice cream. Both husband and wife are good; but somehow not together. They find that they do not love each other any more in the same way they once did. When people are disappointed in marriage because they expect too much, or are disappointed in each other, or have other reasons, they may want to end their marriage. Then they ask a judge to give them a divorce. This is the government's permission to end their marriage.

Some religions have their own laws about divorce. The Catholic religion does not approve of divorce. In the Jewish religion, most Jews require a divorce given by a religious court, a court of rabbis, in addition to the government's permission.

When parents are divorced, they may be angry with each other or they may still be friends. In both cases, the parents, each of them, love the children very much. They still take care of their children. The divorce is not the children's fault; the parents have just stopped loving each other as they once did. But they have not stopped loving their children.

Chapter 13

Not Always—Parents and Children, Brothers and Sisters

We have often said that the love of parents and children for each other is forever. It is natural that it should be. And usually it is. Almost all parents and children love each other more than almost anything else in the whole world.

But not always.

Sometimes the trouble is that children don't understand. They think their parents do not love them—when they really do! Parents may speak to the child in a sharp voice to protect the child from

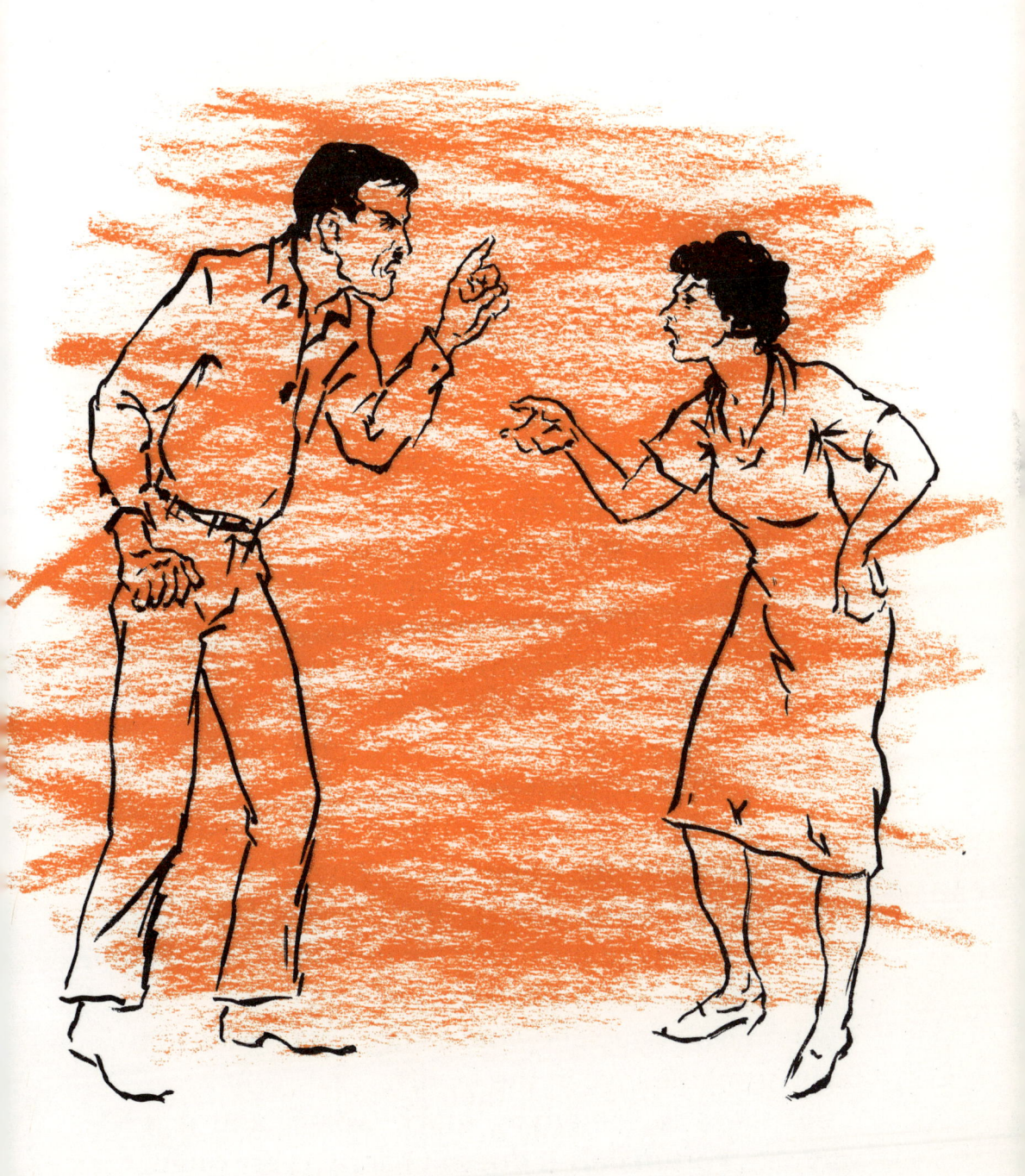

harm. Like "Put that knife down!" Or parents' voices may sound sharp or scolding because they are feeling ill. Or worried. Or angry—at someone else, at themselves, at the world. They are really not scolding the child at all. Parents really love their children much more than the children can understand, until the children themselves grow up and become parents. Then they understand!

Sometimes it is more serious. It is not simply misunderstanding. Even in happy families there are times when a parent gets very angry at a child or a child gets very angry at a parent. Then, in anger, they may say something terrible that they don't really mean. Almost immediately afterwards, they feel sorry for what they said. If they say, "I'm sorry. I didn't really mean that," they both feel better. It helps even if they say it later on. But it helps most if they say it right away.

In most families, now and then, there is some anger and there are some bad feelings. But these feelings are soon over, usually, and easily mended. They are most quickly mended if we say we are angry and explain why. Then we feel better. The hurt isn't deep and doesn't last long. It doesn't really spoil the love in the family.

But there is something much worse, and it is very sad. Fortunately it doesn't happen very often.

There are families where parents and children cannot hold on to the love that is natural for them. Sometimes it is one particular child and one particular parent. Both feel bad about it. Each usually blames the other.

Sometimes a very wise person—perhaps a teacher or counselor, perhaps a rabbi, perhaps a doctor—can help them find out what it is that gets in the way of their love. But sometimes nothing seems to help.

This is one of the saddest things in life, and we would rather it weren't so. Fortunately, it isn't often so. Almost always, the love of parents and children is forever.

Another sad part of life is that sometimes brothers and sisters lose their love for each other. Sometimes they quarrel. At times they may not really understand each other. Or they may be jealous of each other. If they are wise, they will make up quickly. The longer they stay angry, the harder it is to make up. (Here too the first step in making up is to say we are angry and explain why.) But even if they are foolish enough to stay angry for a long time, there still is a deep feeling, underneath the anger, for a brother or sister.

In some cases they never make up and stay angry all through their lives. But more often, even if they are angry for a long time, the deep feeling for each other does not disappear. Family feeling is very strong.

Parents and children usually love each other. So do husbands and wives. And brothers and sisters. And other relatives. And friends. But if we see the world as it really is, and if we are honest, we must add, "but not always."

Chapter 14

Not Always—Adoption

Our bodies work in marvelous ways. One of these is the beginning of a new life, when the life-parts of the husband and the wife, the sperm and the ovum, form the tiny beginning that will become a baby. No wonder the father and the mother are all aglow with love for the new baby! The baby is part of them. It is the joining together of the two of them in a new life. As they cuddle the new baby, they can hardly believe the wonder of it all. It is the "miracle of life."

We have said that the child in the family comes from the joining together of husband and wife. But not always. There are times when a husband and a wife cannot have a child from their own bodies. Our bodies have several different "systems," like our breathing system or our digestive system (which is our eating system). Sometimes one of the systems doesn't work exactly right. Sometimes it is the system that begins a new life that doesn't work exactly right. For this reason, or perhaps for other reasons, the husband and wife do not have a child from their own bodies.

And sometimes, because of the troubles that are part of life, the parents of a baby born in the same way as other babies are not able to care for it.

What happens then? Remember the "magic of love"? The magic of love works not only for husband and wife, who are pulled together in love as though by a magnet. It also makes the two of them, as though they were one, want to give their love, together, to a child.

So the husband and wife who have no child search for a baby whose parents are not able to care for it. And they adopt the baby as their very own. To adopt means to get the government's permission for this child and these parents to belong to each other. It is true that the baby's body comes from other parents. But in every other

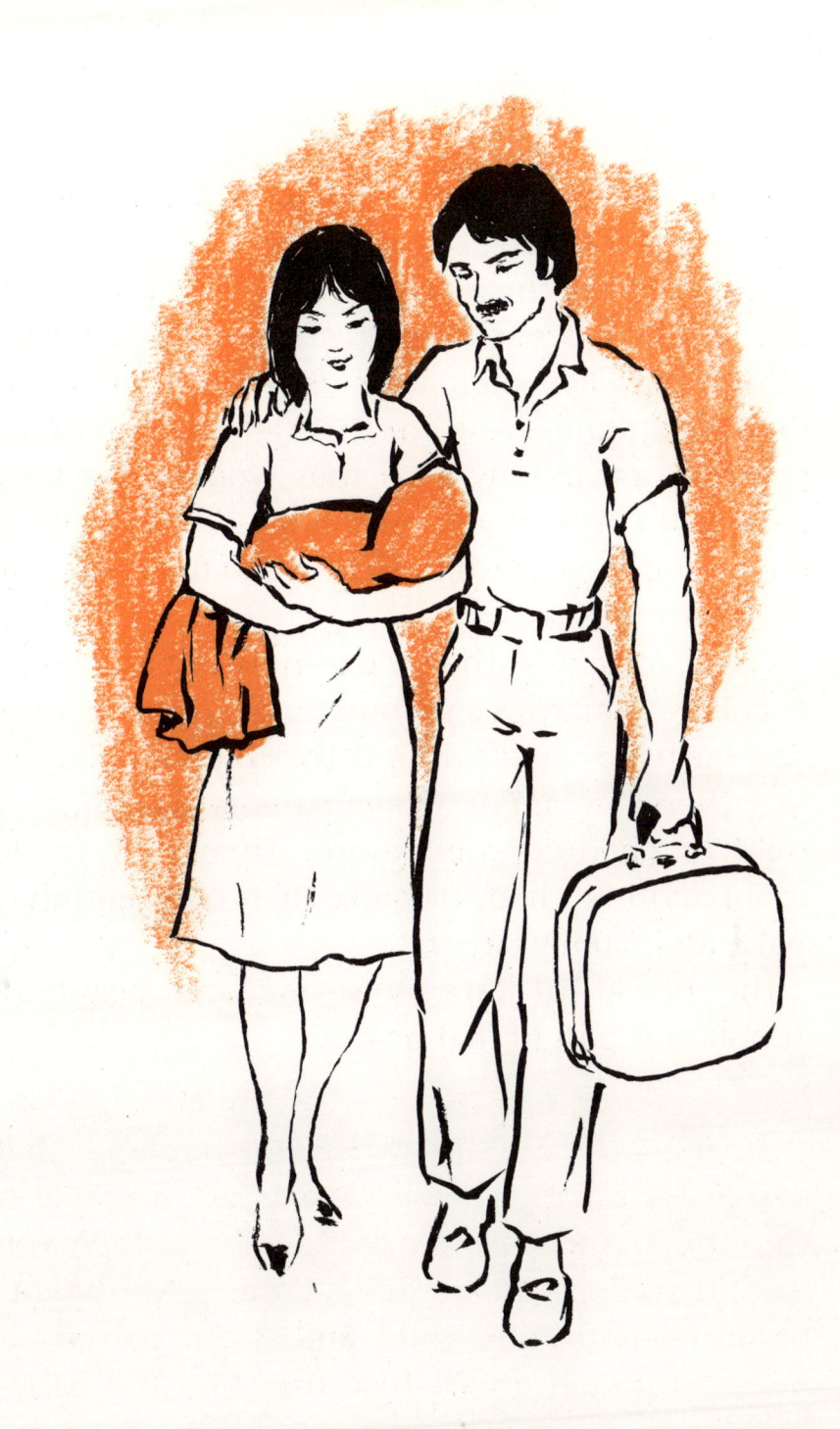

way the adopted baby or child and the parents who adopt it belong to each other.

This is part of the magic of love. The parents and the child love each other. They care for each other. They live their lives as a family, because they are a family. And for their adopted child the parents want exactly what they would want for a child born from their own bodies. The child is theirs, and they give it their love and their care and their lives.

There are times when a parent who has a child, or children, marries a second time. Sometimes the new husband or wife adopts the child or children. And there are times when parents who have a child or children want more. Then they try to adopt another child, or more than one; and they make their family larger.

The power of love is strong and beautiful. Adoption is part of that beauty.

Chapter 15

The Treasures of Our Hearts

What do you think this book has been about? About loving, of course. But the main thing we have been talking about is—What?

What do *you* think we have really been talking about?

Do you remember how this book began? In the earlier chapters we talked about loving God, loving ourselves, our parents, our brothers and sisters, our friends and neighbors. And, yes, loving people whoever they are and wherever they are, even though we don't know them!

All of this is important, and the libraries have many books about each one of these ideas. But none of these ideas is the main reason for *this* book.

This book is about loving too. But the loving we have been talking about, especially, is the love of a man and a woman for each other.

If you are like most people, one day you will marry. Not until you are older, of course, but probably one day you girls will each find a man, and you boys will each find a woman, who becomes very precious to you.

And when you marry that special person, you will probably be doing the most important thing you are likely to do in your whole life!

That is why it is wise to make yourself into the best person you can, so that you will be a very good husband or a very good wife. To help reach this goal it is important to learn to love and respect other people. It is important to respect yourself. And it is important to learn to *give,* even more than to take. When the "magnet" between the sexes begins to work in you, when you are twelve or fourteen or sixteen or whenever, you begin to daydream about the future and about love and marriage. As the years go by, you begin to understand more and more about the world and life and people. Only then will you become grown up

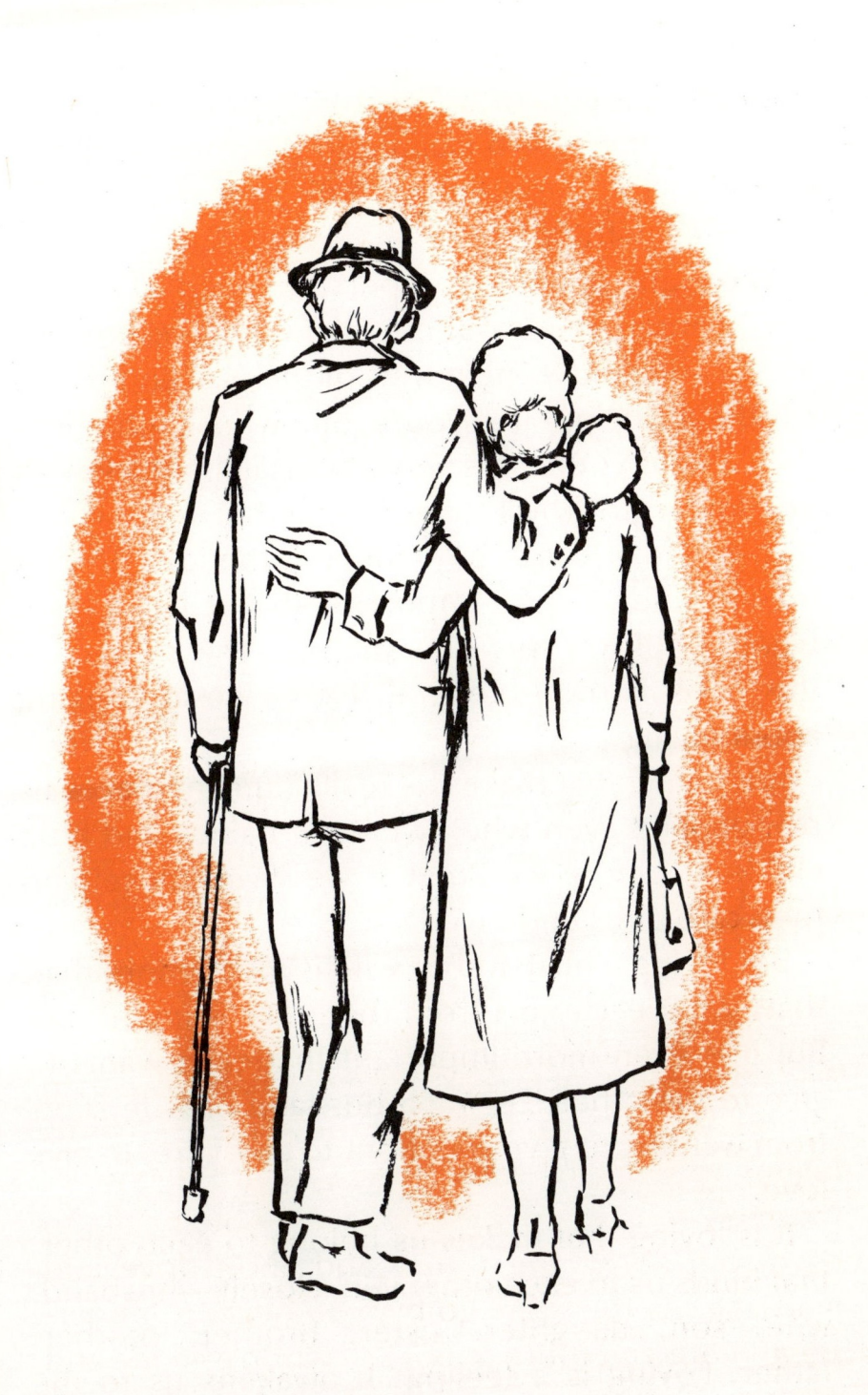

enough, enough of a "person," to be ready for marriage. It is worth waiting to be ready. And it is worth anything to find the right person to marry. Worth everything!

The right person is a person much like you: one whose feelings about life and love are like yours, and whose memories of the past and hopes for the future are like yours, one whose religion is the same as yours. It is very important that a Jewish boy find a girl who is Jewish, and that a girl who is Jewish find a Jewish boy. Indeed, the idea of Jews marrying Jews is so important that it deserves a whole book on this one subject. The subject of this book is more general. Here, we are talking about loving.

It is loving that makes us really human, makes us real people. Even when we were babies and little children, before we knew it we loved those who took care of us and loved us.

But loving a husband or wife is much more than that. What each gets from the other is important. But it is even more important that each wants to *give* to the other. Loving a husband or wife starts from wanting to give affection, to give care, to give love.

It is loving that makes us belong to each other, that binds us to each other very closely—husband, wife, son, daughter, sister, brother, mother, father. Loving is a feeling. It awakens us to the most cherished experiences of our lives, and the happiest. Loving makes us a little like God, for it lets us open wide to others the treasures of our hearts.

One day you will know that some one person has become very precious to you. And, although you are two separate people, you will be able to say to each other, "We two can become one, for our love makes my heart yours and yours mine."

A husband and wife who truly love each other have found great treasure. If they are wise and appreciate it, they will guard it carefully and protect it from being lost or spoiled or stolen. A man and a woman who love each other deeply want to keep their treasure safe and strong, forever glowing, forever bright.